Nutribullet Recipes

Lose Weight, Fight Aging, Gain Energy, and Improve Overall Health with the Superfood Detox Cleanse Smoothies

By:

J.J. Lewis

Want more Bestseller Cook Books for FREE?

Join my **V.I.P** Reading List where I give away **Healthy** and Delicious Recipes FOR **FREE!**

Yes, you heard me right! COMPLETELY FREE to everyone just for being a loyal reader of mine!

http://www.mritchi.com/freecookbook

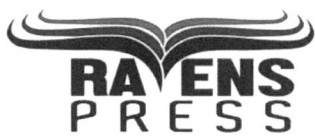

ISBN-13: 978-1514785966

ISBN-10: 151478596X

www.amazon.com/author/jjlewis

Contents

Introduction

Nutribullet is a widely popular super food extractor that can help you achieve your health and fitness goals. The patented technology in Nutribullet will enable you to prepare high quality smoothies, soups, and many other healthy meals easily.

Each drink and dish in this recipe book is guaranteed to come out smooth and creamy yet retain the pulp for fiber content, as long as you use the Nutribullet correctly. Choose from a variety of energy smoothies that you can drink first thing in the morning, green smoothies to help you get your daily amount of vegetables, detox smoothies to help cleanse and revitalize your digestive system, and soups that will keep you satiated and well-nourished. You will also be happy to know that there are also bonus recipes that will show you how to make dips, spreads, and condiments.

Bring out the full potential of your Nutribullet and maximize its amazing features. You will soon discover how easy it actually is to prepare tasty and healthy drinks and dishes within the comforts of your own home.

Thanks again for downloading this book, I hope you enjoy it!

C H A P T E R   1
The Nutribullet in your Kitchen

It seems that everyone nowadays lives such busy lives that they tend to turn to quick and easy meal solutions in order to stay sane. Well, this may be the reason why smoothies are immensely popular among urban households. Smoothies take only a few minutes to prepare and are much healthier compared to microwave meals and fast food.

However, what a lot of people do not know is that the blender plays a crucial role in properly extracting nutrients from the ingredients. Cheap and low quality blenders tend to expose the delicate fruits, vegetables, and other ingredients to a certain level of heat that it ends up destroying most of the nutrients. You then end up consuming a much lower amount of nutrients than what you bargained for.

It is important to invest instead in a blender that will not only make it easy for you to process your smoothies but also contribute to retaining the best nutritional value from your chosen ingredients. The Nutribullet is one such blender that is reputed to have helped thousands of people from all over the world make smoothies that have helped them lose weight, gain energy, and improve their overall health.

How the Nutribullet Works

The Nutribullet, which is marketed as "The Superfood Extractor" is designed to do just that: it breaks down the ingredients by pulverizing it all to make the smoothest possible smoothie. This extraction process will make it easier for your body to absorb the nutrients from the ingredients and quickly distribute it throughout your cells.

The Nutribullet works on a powerful 600-watt motor and with what is called the "Extractor" blades (which are actually patented, by the way) that are sharp enough to completely break down even the hardest of root vegetables, nuts, stems, and seeds. The motor applies a so called "cyclonic action" that easily pulverizes the ingredients, including ice, without you having to shake or poke at the mixture every now and then.

Nutribullet has three types of blades that you can choose from depending on your needs. For instance, crushing ice and turning nuts, seeds, and grains into flour require different blades compared to the one that you will use for smoothies alone.

One major advantage of owning a Nutribullet is that it is so compact to the point of being portable. It can be stored quite easily because of its shape and size, despite the fact that you can blend up to 24 ounces of ingredients. Also, apart from smoothies, it can be used to mill nuts, grains, and seeds into meal, flour, and butter.

Another thing to be happy about the Nutribullet is that its cups are BPA-free, which means that the cups do not contain the toxic chemical called phthalates. However, since the cups still contain plastic, you must remember to never pour anything hot or even warm inside the cups. For hot soup recipes, let the soup cool down to room temperature completely first before pouring it into the Nutribullet cup cup, then heat up the soup again after blending.

The Proper Way to Use your Nutribullet

There are three pieces which constitute the Nutribullet: the first is the base which holds the processor engine, the second piece is the tops that contain the blade attachment, and the last is a "bullet" shaped (conical and oval) glass cup.

To use the Nutribullet safely and effectively, you start by placing the ingredients into the cup, attach the blade attachment on top not unlike a lid to a jar, and then start blending. Take note that you should never go beyond the "MAX" line of the cup when you are filling it up with ingredients. Going beyond this line will cause the ingredients to overflow and cause a mess that you will have to spend more time cleaning up than preparing your smoothies.

To transfer the smoothie from the blender, simply remove the cup from the processor, turn it upside down, detach the blade attachment, and pour the smoothie from the cup to your glass.

Once you have finished using your Nutribullet, you can easily clean it by following any one of the two tips. The first method is to detach the blade attachment and cup and rinse them in a basin of water, and then place them in the dishwasher. The second is by pouring soapy water into the cup and connecting it back to the blade attachment. Run the blender very quickly, then rinse and set aside to dry. Make sure that any residue is rinsed off thoroughly; otherwise, any trapped bits of ingredients will contaminate your next smoothie.

C H A P T E R   2

Important Guidelines for Nutriblast Preparation

Nutriblast is the term for foods that you have prepared using the Nutribullet. To make sure that your Nutriblast smoothies and soups will retain maximum nutritional value and flavor, keep in mind the following guidelines:

On Making Chilled Smoothies:

Ice cubes are often used in smoothies, but if you really want to amp up the nutritional value of your Nutriblast smoothies, then you should use frozen fruit instead. After all, ice cubes can cause the smoothies to be a bit watered down and not as flavorful, which is why people traditionally add sugar to their smoothies.

To freeze your fruit, simply place them, whole and unpeeled, in the freezer. For fruits that have already been peeled and/or sliced, put them in freezer bags before placing them in the freezer, making sure that as much of the air inside of the bag is pressed out before sealing. Fruits which are easiest to freeze and slice are pineapples, bananas, and melons. Other fruits might require you to attach the Nutribullet cup blade that is specifically designed to crush ice.

On Fast and Easy Blending:

Even though the Nutribullet is designed for emulsifying tough ingredients, it is still a good idea to chop up your fruits, vegetables, and nuts so that it will be much faster to blend. Doing so will also extend the life of your Nutribullet blades.

It is generally not recommended to chop your ingredients beforehand because this will expose the delicate nutrients stored inside and cause them to oxidize. However, if you want to do slice your fruits and vegetables the night before blending them, then store them in resealable plastic bags and push as much air out of the bag before closing. Follow the procedure on how to chill fruit after that.

On Choosing Ingredients:

Always go for fresh and organic ingredients and as often as possible, stick to locally grown and in-season products. Organic ingredients do not contain harmful toxins from fertilizers and pesticides, and since you will be blending your ingredients raw, you certainly would not want any of those substances to get into your body.

It is also imperative for you to have a variety of ingredients. Use the natural color of produce as a general guide on where you can get different nutrients.

For instance, red fruits and vegetables, such as tomatoes and red bell peppers, contain lycopene, which is a very potent antioxidant that helps keep the heart and brain healthy.

Green produce such as broccoli, spinach, and kale are rich in chlorophyll, which is essential for healthy eyes, teeth, and bones. The phytochemicals in leafy greens have strong anti-cancer properties as well.

Tan and white produce such as bananas and garlic contain allicin, which has natural antibacterial and antiviral properties. Your immune system will be boosted greatly.

Yellow and orange fruits and vegetables are rich in carotenoids, which are essential to the eyes and immune system. Make sure to add carrots and pumpkin to your smoothies and soups.

Purple and blue produce are very rich in antioxidants, particularly anthocyanin, which helps keep skin, hair, and nails strong and healthy. This antioxidant also helps minimize inflammation.

On Storing Smoothies:

Always remember that you should drink your smoothie as soon as you have finished blending it. The reason for this is that once the nutrients have been released from the ingredients, they easily get destroyed due to oxidation. Therefore you must only blend if you are certain that you will drink the smoothie right after.

However, if you really want to blend your smoothie now and drink it later, or slowly while on the go, what you can do is add a tablespoon of lemon juice to your smoothie. The vitamin C in the lemon juice will help prevent oxidation for a short while. Mind you, adding lemon juice will change the flavor of the smoothie. Apart from adding lemon juice, you should also pour the smoothie into a glass container with a tight lid, such as a mason jar. Then, refrigerate until you are ready to drink.

On Drinking Green Smoothies:

It is recommended that everyone should eat about three servings of vegetables every day. Unfortunately, most people who follow the traditional Western diet barely eat any vegetables at all.

You must make it a point to prepare at least 8 ounces of green smooth and consume it each day. For those of you how want to lose weight, you must drink 64 ounces of green smoothie. Additionally, mix in flax seeds or chia seeds in your green smoothies to further promote weight loss.

Try to use two or more leafy green vegetables in each smoothie, because varying the kinds of greens that you will use will also minimize the level of alkaloids (or the nitrogen in plants) that you consume.

Health benefits of smoothies:

We live in a very fast moving world where we don't even spare time for our families let alone for maintaining our health. Most of the people 'fuel' themselves using junk food like hamburgers, pizzas, burritos, etc. How can they expect to gain all the necessary vitamins and minerals through these things? For such people, smoothies are the most viable option. They can be made instantly and you can have them quickly before doing whatever it is that you do.

Necessary Vitamins and Minerals:

Vitamins and minerals are essential for the human body. The most common sources are seasonal fruits and vegetables but people generally do not eat these things on a daily basis.

Vital elements like vitamin C, folate and potassium can be obtained from citrus fruits like oranges, lemons and from tropical fruits which include papaya, pineapple, avocados, coconut, pomegranates, bananas and mangoes. These fruits are widely used in smoothies because they taste good and they provide you with numerous health benefits. These fruits are the main ingredients of the recipes included in this book.

Vitamin C is known to boost up the immune system by helping in the synthesis of collagen, a protein that forms blood clots, muscular and arterial structures and ligaments. Potassium on the other hand is crucial for healthy functioning of heart muscles and regulating blood pressure. It also prevents the formation of oxalic acid, a nasty compound that causes kidney stones.

Folate is also a very important element that enhances cellular health and repairs the worn out tissues of the body. Some of the above mentioned fruits are also rich in manganese and beta carotene. Magnesium is very important for our skeletal structures, nerves and thyroid glands. Beta carotene is crucial for eyes and it boosts up the natural defense of our body against bacteria and viruses.

Fiber:

For those of you who don't know the importance of fiber; let me tell you that you simply can't digest your food without it. An average person requires about 25 to 38 grams of fiber per day depending upon the age and sex. Well, if you are facing problems like constipation, weight gain, high blood and sugar levels and nausea, then you seriously need to get yourself a load of fiber. And what better way to do so than by having a yummy fruit or green smoothie. Your preference should be to try smoothies that are composed of blackberries, pears, apples, melons, celery, kale or beet leaves.

Water:

"Water is life." This quote is true to its core. Your body would simply cease to function properly due to the lack of water. Drinking fruit or green smoothies is a good way not only to stay hydrated but also to fulfill your nutritional requirements. Your blood flow will remain normal, thus saving you from problems like high blood pressure and formation of clots in the blood vessels. Also, your excretion mechanisms will work effectively and you won't have to face problems like constipation, kidney stones, bladder infections, etc. It is said that staying hydrated slows down aging so you should definitely try these smoothies. Who knows you might actually live longer and healthier.

Antioxidants:

Antioxidants are crucial for one's health. If you want to stay away from cancers, heart problems, DNA degeneration and several common diseases, then your diet must have an adequate quantity of antioxidants. Lucky for you, my smoothie recipes are solely comprised of fruits and vegetables that are rich in antioxidant minerals.

The most common antioxidants are macro-minerals like magnesium, calcium, sodium, potassium, sulfur, phosphorus, etc. Other types of antioxidants are vitamins C and E. All of these minerals and vitamins are abundant in fresh green vegetables like kale, celery, spinach, cucumber and in tropical and citrus fruits like blueberries, raspberries, oranges, strawberries, mangoes, avocados, coconut, etc.

CHAPTER 3

The Ingredient Guide for Nutribullet Recipe

To make smoothies that are guaranteed to jump-start your day and help you achieve your long term fitness goals, you must put a lot of effort into choosing the right ingredients. These ingredients are scientifically proven to contain essential vitamins, minerals, fats, amino acids, and antioxidants that will nourish and revitalize your cells.

A List of Nutrients to Know

The essential vitamins that your body needs are the following: Vitamins A, B1 or Thiamin, B2 or Riboflavin, B3 or Niacin, B4 or Choline/ Adenine, B5 or Pantothenic Acid, B6 or Pyridoxines, B7 or Biotin, B9 or Folates, B12 or Cobalamin, and C, D3, E, and K.

The essential minerals are calcium, copper, iron, phosphorus, magnesium, manganese, selenium potassium, sodium, and zinc.

The essential fats are the omega 3 fatty acids that can be derived from vegetables, nuts, and seeds.

The essential amino acids are namely: Tryptophan, Tyrosine, Threonine, Isoleucine, Histidine, Leucine, Lysine, Methionine, Phenylaneline, Cysteine, and Valine.

Daily consumption of a combination of these essential nutrients will keep you fit and full of energy. These benefits include:

Stronger immune system; higher resistance to viral and bacterial infections

Lower risk of developing cancer, type 2 diabetes, osteoporosis, Alzheimer's and other degenerative diseases

Improved cardiovascular health

Healthy digestive system, including regular bowel movement

Alleviation of symptoms such as PMS, inflammation, and allergies

Regulation of blood sugar and cholesterol level

Suggested Ingredients for Energy Smoothies

Stock up your fridge with these high energy ingredients that you can blend any time using your Nutribullet. Energy smoothies are best served in the morning to give you that extra boost to jump-start your day. Of course, that does not mean you cannot enjoy it later on as well. Here is a list of ingredients:

Fruits: Bananas, Citrus fruits (grapefruit, lemon, lime, orange, kiwi), Berries (strawberries, blueberries, blackberries, raspberries, etc), Apples, Pineapple, Papaya

Vegetables: Spinach, Bell peppers, Sweet potato

Liquid Base: coconut water, milk (dairy, almond, hemp, rice, oat, soy, coconut, hazelnut, etc), Tea, Juices

Others: Honey, Almonds, Yogurt, Beans, Nuts, Seeds

Suggested Ingredients for Green Smoothies

Try out all of the green smoothie recipes in this book, and if you feel that you have tasted them all and would like to have something new, then mix and match the following recommended ingredients. Do not be afraid to experiment and always prioritize organic, locally produced, and in season produce.

Fruit: banana, mango, grape, pineapple, grapefruit, peach, lime, lemon, apple (Fuji and green), kiwi, apricot, papaya, cantaloupe

Greens: Broccoli, Kale, Cucumber, Mint, Collard Greens, Spinach, Fennel, Swiss Chard, Parsley, Baby Beet Greens, Cabbage, Lettuce, Endives, Zucchini, Purslane, Dandelion Greens, Garden Cress

Liquid Base: Coconut water, Filtered water, Milk and Yogurt (dairy, almond, hemp, rice, oat, soy, coconut, hazelnut, etc), Tea (green, mint, white, yerba mate), Juices (apple, orange, pineapple, grapefruit, etc)

Others: avocado, Oats, Coconut, Cocoa powder, Seeds (hemp, chia, sunflower flax), Rice bran, Walnuts, Pecans, Almonds, Wheat germ, Ginger, Cinnamon

Suggested Ingredients for Detox Smoothies

It is never a bad idea to give your body a break from eating foods that are difficult to digest and may cause sluggishness. That is why it is best for you to detoxify every now and then. This little habit can become easier with a Nutribullet and the recipes in this book. You can also whip up your own detox drink using these ingredients:

Fruit: Berries (blueberries, blackberries, raspberries), Apricots, Lemon, Avocado, Grapefruit

Vegetables: Tomatoes, Arugula, Watercress, Cabbage, Green Pepper, Artichokes, Asparagus, Beet, Broccoli, Kale

Others: Coconut, Ginger, Sesame Seeds, Dandelion, Green tea, Lemon grass, Olive oil, Seaweed, Wheat grass

MUST READ: Caution on Ingredients

There are certain guidelines that you must never forget. The first is to always remove the stones and pips of the following fruits: cherry, plum, pear, apricot, peach, and apple. The stones and pips of these fruits contain cyanide, a deadly poison.

Next, take not that there are certain things that you should never eat raw. One is the rhubarb leaves, because eating them raw will trigger convulsions, kidney stones, and comes. Another thing that you need to avoid are tomato vines and leaves. While tomatoes are perfectly alright eaten raw, its greens contain poisons that will trigger severe nausea.

Lastly, never eat raw beans such as Lima beans and kidney beans. Consuming them raw will poison you.

So, are you ready to start using your Nutribullet? Keep in mind that all the recipes in this book will give you 1 to 2 servings each. If you are planning to fill more glasses or bowls than that, then simple double up the amount of servings.

C H A P T E R 4
Smoothie Recipes for a Healthy Heart

Health problems are increasing every year, thanks to fast food and unhealthy lifestyles. But there is still an easy and tasty way to overcome this problem and to keep your heart healthy, happy and loving. It's not hard like exercise, and it is also not yucky like medicines. Dropping the curtains…here are some yummy smoothie recipes that'll keep your heart healthy. You just have to grab some fruits and vegetables and blend them.

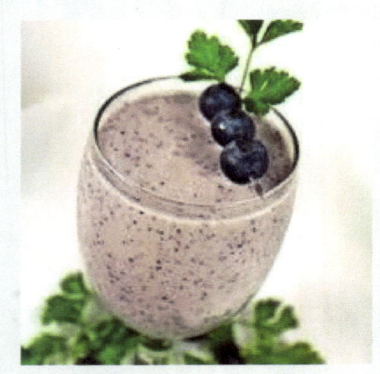

Ingredients

Avocado – 1/4

Blueberries – 1 cup

Lime juice (half lemon)

Coconut water – 1 cup

Honey – 1 Tbsp

1. Avocado and Blueberry Smoothie

This smoothie recipe should be your number on choice because it is packed with disease fightin phytochemicals and anti-oxidants from blueberries an it also provides you with monounsaturated fatty acid which are the 'good' fats. Avocados are rich in thes 'good' fats and they are famous for lowering LDI which is the 'bad' cholesterol and it increases the leve of HDL which is the 'good' cholesterol. Aside fror this talk of good and bad cholesterol, avocados are good source of vitamin B-6 and folic acid which to provide good heart support.

Blend until it is nice and smooth.

2. Acai Berry and Chia Seed Smoothie

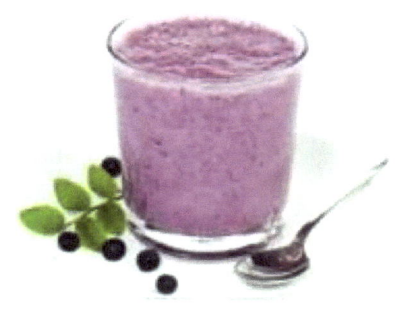

Ingredients

Frozen Acai berries – 3.5 ounces

Chia seeds – 2 Tbs.

Unsweetened almond milk – 2 cups

Liquid stevia – to taste

Acai seeds can be easily purchased in the form of frozen packets from any drug store. They too are rich in anti-oxidants just like a heart-friendly food. They are also helpful in preventing atherosclerosis. Chia seeds are also good for heart health because they help in reducing blood pressure. Omega-3 fatty acids in chia seeds are useful for keeping your heart healthy.

First, blend milk and berries at low speed to brea down the berries. Then blend the mixture at high spee until it is smooth. After that, add chia seeds and stevi; Adjust the sweetness according to your taste.

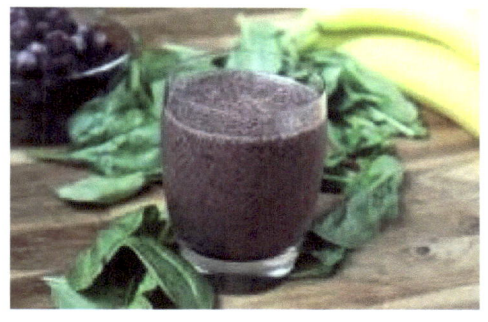

Ingredients

Hemp protein powder – 4 Tbs.

Almond milk – 1 cup

Berries – half cup

1 banana

1 handful spinach

Blend properly and enjoy.

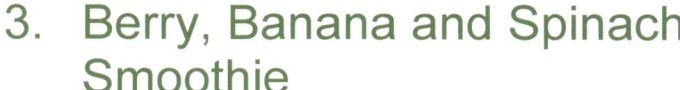

3. Berry, Banana and Spinach Smoothie

Berries are very nutritious and they have anti-oxidant which as we all know are essential for a healthy hear Banana is a great source of potassium which keep blood pressure in control and spinach has somethin called Co-Q10 which is useful in the prevention an treatment of cardiovascular disease. Hemp is a goo ingredient to improve cardiovascular health.

4. Green Lemonade

This green lemonade is a must try because it offers a great many benefits to your heart. Apples contain compounds that delay the breakdown of LDL i.e. bad cholesterol. Lemons help in boosting the immune system and reducing weight. Since obesity

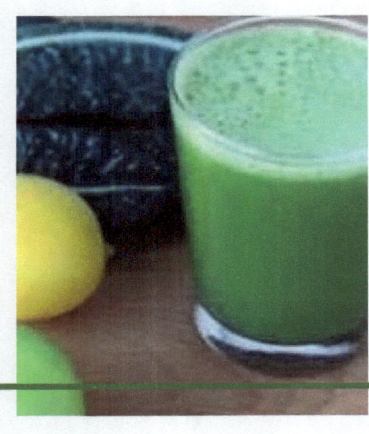

Ingredients

2 green apples

1 handful of   greens

A half peeled   lemon

is one of the major causes of heart diseases, lemons are great for this purpose. Greens such as spinach, mint, kale, collard, coriander, chard etc. are also said to be really beneficial for the heart, especially spinach because it is rich in potassium, iron, fiber, lutein and folate.

Blend all ingredients and drink immediately.

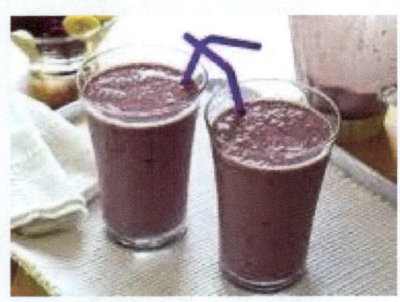

Ingredients

Skim milk – half cup

Nonfat yoghurt – half cup

1 banana

Raspberries – half cup

Almond butter – 1 Tbs.

Sweetened dark cocoa powder – 1 Tbsp

3 ice cubes

5. Heart-Friendly Smoothie

Potassium and calcium in milk and yoghurt help in reducing weight by making you feel full and satisfied. These elements also help in lowering blood pressure. Cocoa beans are also good for promoting a healthy heart circulation as they contain flavanol. Last but not least, almonds increase the level of HDL and reduce the level of LDL. Hmmm…This really is a heart-friendly smoothie. An interesting name for a smoothie, isn't it?

Combine them in your Nutribullet and blend them wel

6. Fruit Smoothie

Everyone likes fruits and if combined together, they are mouth-watering. Oranges, bananas, berries, papaya and grapes makes a sensational smoothie. Besides taste, fruits are good for your heart's health due to a treasure reserve of healthy elements present in them.

Place all these amazing ingredients in your Nutribulle blend and enjoy!

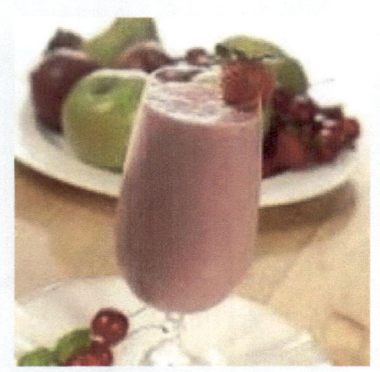

Ingredients

1 banana

1 cup blueberries

1 papaya

1 cup red grape juice

1 cup orange juice

1 cup carrot juice

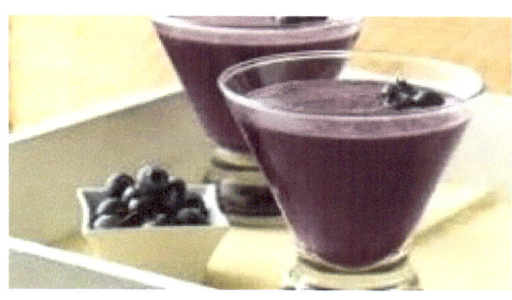

Ingredients

Pure pomegranate juice – half cup

Unsweetened, frozen berries – 3/4 cup

Lemon zest – 1/2 teaspoon

Fresh lemon juice – 1/2 teaspoon

Nonfat vanilla yoghurt – 1/4 cup

3 to 4 ice cubes

7. Pomegranate-Blueberry Smoothie

Pomegranate has such a bright and beautiful color like some precious stones. It is one of the best fruits to keep you healthy and to cure your diseases. It is a very powerful anti-oxidant just like blueberries. It restrains abnormal platelet growth to reduce cardiac and stroke risks and it also reduces cholesterol and blood pressure.

First, add all the ingredients except ice. Blend unt they are smooth. Then add the ice cubes and blen until it is crushed and looks yummy. Enjoy thi splendid drink.

CHAPTER 5

Appetizing Detox Smoothies

Don't make a face like that! Yeah…the little frowns over there…yes, good because you have no need to pinch your nose while drinking these delectable detox smoothies. That's right! These are some of the most delicious yet very healthy detox smoothie recipes. They are packed with anti-oxidants which neutralize free radicals and cleanse your body. So, experience the richness and flavor of all the ingredients while you give your body what it needs. There you go with some super-dooper recipes.

1. Happy Berry Breakfast

Enjoy this wonderful detox smoothie which is packed with a punch of anti-oxidants! Oh! And honey will purify your body from the inside out, giving your skin a nice glow.

Combine them all in a blender. Blend and enjoy.

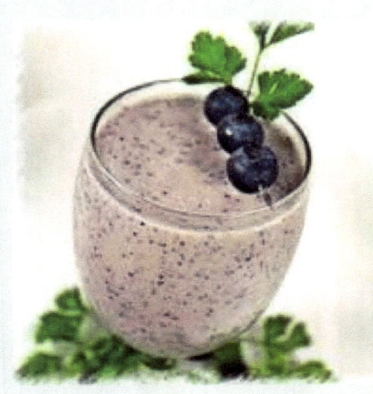

Ingredients

Unsweetened, frozen raspberries – 1 cup

Frozen unsweetened cherries – 1/4 cup

Freshly grated ginger – 2 tsp

Unsweetened, chilled almond milk – 3/4 cup

Honey – 1 Tbsp

Fresh lemon juice – 2 tsp

Ground flaxseed – 1 tsp

2. Green Smoothie

Greens are full of iron and elements that wipe out all the toxics from your body. Plus they are rich in fiber which eliminates all the chances of constipation. You will feel really good if you try this recipe.

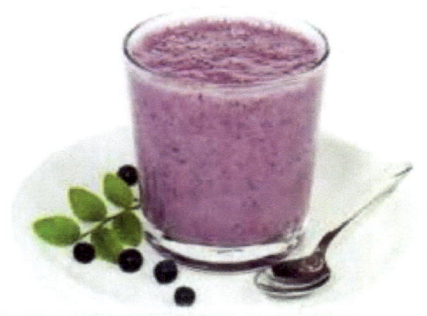

Ingredients

Chopped kale leaves – 1/4 cup

Mango cubes – 1 cup

2 chopped medium ribbed celery

Fresh orange juice – 1 cup

Fresh chopped mint – 1/4 cup

Chopped parsley – 1/4 cup

Blend them nice and smooth and have a drink.

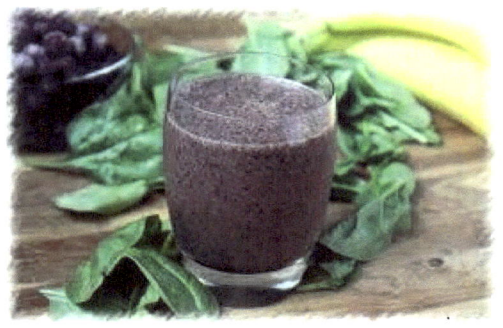

Ingredients

Kale – 1 cup

Half pear

1/4 avocado

Half lemon

Half cucumber

Coconut water – half cup

Ginger – half inch

1 scoop protein powder (pea, pumpkin or hemp)

Water

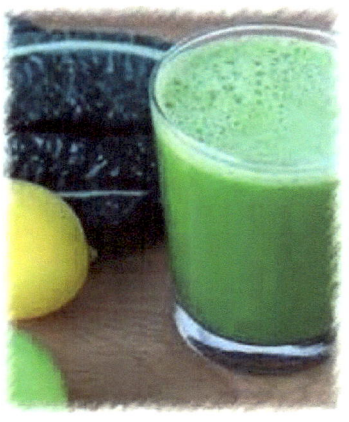

Ingredients

Half pear

1 cup spinach

1/4 avocado

1 cup almond milk

1/4 cup coconut water

3. Kale Smoothie

Kale and ginger, a great combination! Ginger is good for digestion and kale has all the qualities which are possessed by green vegetables.

Blend them and there you have a healthy drink.

4. Alkalinity Delight

As you can see from the name, this recipe will neutralize the acidity in the stomach and give you a really soothing feeling.

Blend them well.

1 scoop protein powder

1 teaspoon chia seeds

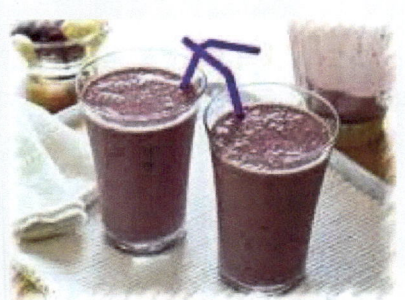

Ingredients

Papaya – 1 cup

Juice from a half lime

Coconut kefir – 1 cup

Raw honey – 1 Tbsp

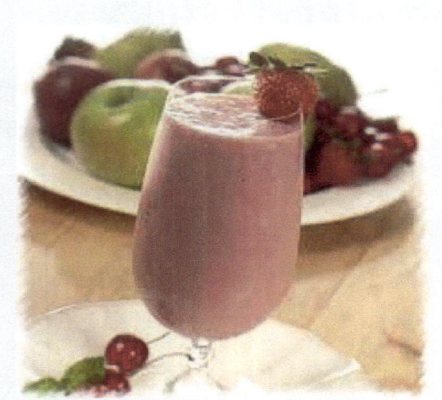

Ingredients

Jicama – half cup

5 romaine lettuce leaves

Half cucumber

1/4 avocado

A handful of cilantro

1 date

Hemp protein – 4 scoops

1 whole lime

5. Papaya Smoothie

Papayas are rich in vitamins C and E. These vitamins and coconut kefir together make a good detox smoothie. Coconut kefir has a healthy dose of probiotics which are good for your stomach.

Such an easy recipe! Blend them and sooth your belly with this light smoothie.

6. Smooth Vitamin C and Fiber

This recipe contains a root vegetable called jicama which is rich in vitamin C.

Blend well.

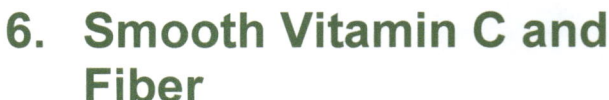

7. Morning Freshness

If you make cucumber the base of your detox

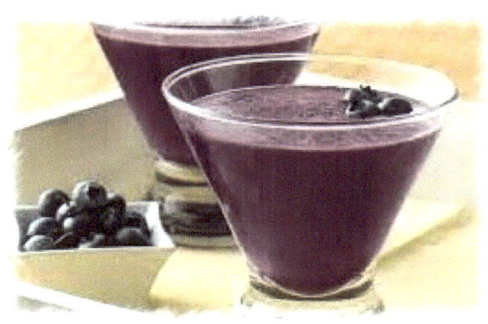

smoothie, it's a wise choice. It not only hydrates your body but it is also alkaline in nature. It provides you with some minerals as well.

Wash and cut all ingredients. After that, make a nice juice/shake and freshen up yourself.

Ingredients

1 cucumber

2 stalks of celery

A fistful of romaine

A fistful of kale

1 green apple

1 broccoli stem

Half peeled lemon

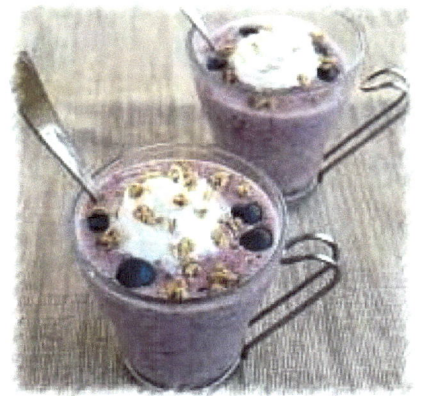

8. Cranberry Smoothie

Try this brilliant cranberry smoothie not only to detox your body but also to keep your kidneys strong. It is rich in vitamin C, E, K, manganese and a large number of phytonutrients which keeps you miles and miles away from urinary tract infection, cardiovascular disease, cancer and dental problems. Say hello to this remarkable smoothie!

Juice them all and take advantage of this very healthy smoothie.

Ingredients

Cranberries – half cup

1 cucumber

1 pear

1 apple

1 celery stalk

A handful of spinach

C H A P T E R   6

Smoothie Recipes for Improved Energy

If you need to boost your energy, smoothies are a great and instant way of doing that. Don't go for coffee, tea or an artificial energy drink to give you a kick start. Instead go for the healthier options like a nourishing glass of smoothie. In the presence of such energy boosting smoothies you need not worry about your weakening immune system. They are rich in carbohydrates, proteins, calcium, vitamins, minerals and a lot more to increase the energy reserves of your body.

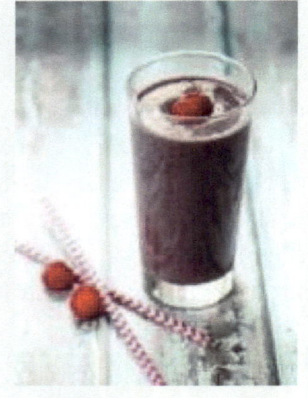

Ingredients

Fresh tangerine juice of 3 tangerines

A handful of frozen strawberries

Fresh juice of a red grapefruit

1. Fresh Morning Smoothie

Vitamin C, anti-oxidants, carbohydrates and great flavor are what make this an ideal morning smoothie.

Mix the strawberries with the juice of tangerines and grapefruit and blend the mixture. This delicious and very easy recipe will bring a smile to your face. Gotta try it!

2. Blueberry-Mango Smoothie

Blueberry is a wonderful source of anti-oxidants and mango is the king. Mangoes are a good source of

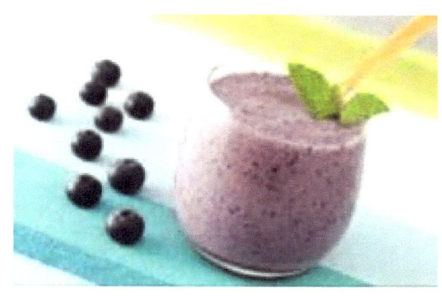

Ingredients

1 pint of blueberries

1 mango

1 banana

1 cup of almond milk

1 tsp of maple syrup

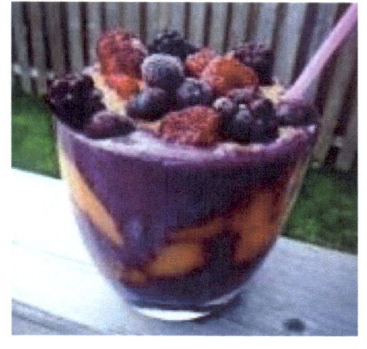

Ingredients

Blueberries – half cup

Blackberries – half cup

Cherries – half cup

1 banana

Honey – 1 tsp

Almond milk – 1 cup

Flaxseed oil – 1 Tbsp

Dash of cinnamon

Caretenoids and vitamin C which help in boosting the immune system. Apart from these advantages, this smoothie contains bananas which are known to be an instant source of energy.

Chop the mangoes and then blend all the ingredients in a blender. Your energizing drink is ready. Add some ice if you like.

3. Berry Berry

Berries are popular in smoothies not just because they look good and they taste good but because they have so much more to offer in terms of improving your health. They have disease fighting phytochemicals, specifically blueberries. Berries are also a rich source of anti-oxidants, as mentioned time and again. Honey is also an important energy boosting ingredient, sweet but way better than the processed sugar.

Blend them until you see the smooth and creamy texture.

4. Strawberry Smoothie

Strawberries boost immunity! How? They are an excellent source of vitamin C which is a well-known immunity booster and also a great anti-oxidant. You can get your daily requirement of Vitamin C from this smoothie.

Puree them in your blender and get your much needed vitamin C.

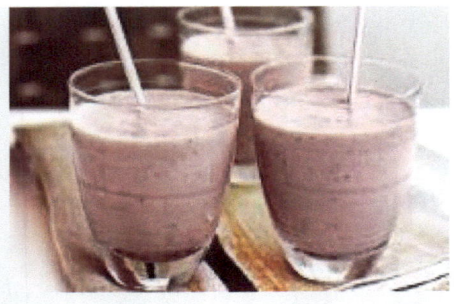

Ingredients

Strawberries – 1 cup

1 sliced frozen banana

Coconut milk – 1 cup

Honey – 1 tsp

5. Peach Smoothie

Peaches combat diseases including cancer and they also lower the risk of heart diseases. They give you an amazing boost of energy and nourish your skin as well.

Peel and chop the peach and pop all the ingredients in your blender. Now what? Grab a glass and drink.

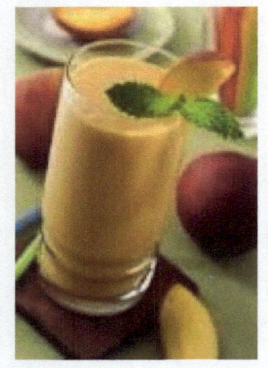

Ingredients

1 peach

Strawberries / raspberries – half cup

Low fat peach yoghurt – half cup

Milk – 1/4 cup

6. Melon Smoothie

Dehydrated after exercise or some tough physical work? This melon smoothie will hydrate you as water melon contains 92% water and make you feel fresh again.

Blend them until it is smooth and freshen up with this rich drink.

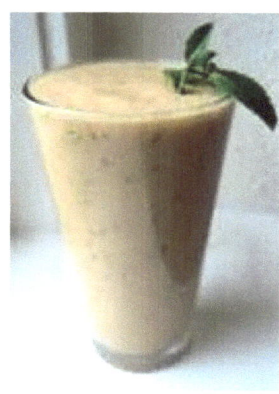

Ingredients

Watermelon cubes – 1 cup

Honeydew melon cubes – half cup

Cantaloupe cubes – 1 cup

Frozen strawberries – 1 cup

7. Fruit Luxury

Fruits provide you with all the energy if you cut on your diet to reduce weight. You won't feel weak and you will not gain weight if you try this smoothie recipe. This smoothie is made of pineapples, oranges, berries and bananas. Combine all the benefits and you get a wonderful source of energy.

Peel and section the oranges. Juice the oranges and pineapple and add water. Then add all the ingredients. Start on low speed to crush the ice and then speed up to make a smooth drink. You will feel like you are on a beach enjoying a nice and refreshing drink.

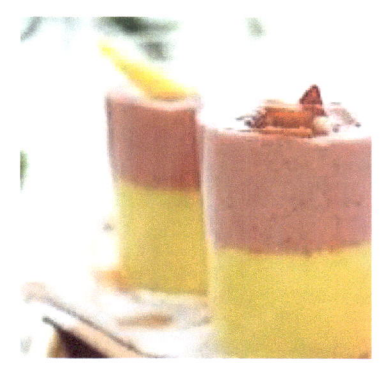

Ingredients

5 slices of pineapple

1 banana

2 oranges

A handful of berries

1/4 cup of water

Some ice

8. Kiwi Smoothie

Kiwi is also one of the keys to boost your immune system because it contains twice the amount of vitamin C that oranges do. It is also a good source of potassium which will keep your heart healthy and strong. This recipe has two more ingredients which will give strength to your immune system, mangoes and the algae called Spirulina. So, this recipe will give you 3 times more energy than eating a single fruit.

Peel and chop mango and kiwis. Add into the blender along with the coconut milk. Blend until the fruit is mixed. Then add the rest of the ingredients and keep the machine on until it is smooth. Add some ice and drink to your heart's delight.

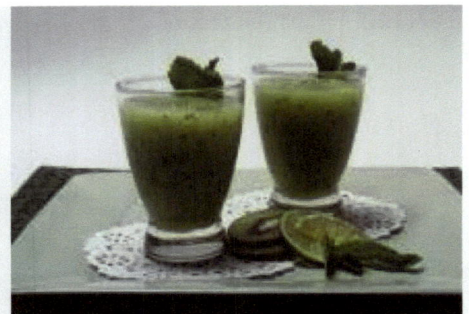

Ingredients

2 kiwis

1 mango

2 tsp Spirulina powder

100 ml of coconut milk

2 tsp honey

75 ml of low fat yoghurt

C H A P T E R   7

Smoothie Recipes for Beautiful Skin

Are you tired of using different kinds of skin freshness creams and lotions that still haven't produced your desired results? If yes, then throw those useless things out the window right away and go for something that really works. I'm talking about yummy smoothies made of fresh fruits and vegetables. The amount of skin freshening nutrients in these recipes is enormous.

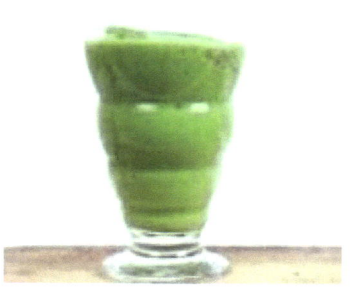

Ingredients

4 lettuce leaves

1 baby kale

4 sprays of parsley

A small lemon

A Fuji apple

A banana

2 TB of flax seeds mixed with chia seeds

Half a glass of water

4 ice cubes

1/16 table spoon of stevia

1. The Green Beauty Smoothie

Lettuce, parsley and apples with bananas and kale is a conventional yet exceedingly enticing recipe that will make you feel lighter. The cleansing agents in these ingredients will take good care of your skin.

Add kale, romaine, apple, parsley, lemon, cucumber, ginger, and water to your blender. After that close the lid and switch on your blender. The contents will be broken down in about 15-20 seconds. Then add the remaining ingredients to the blender. Blend the mixture for 1 minute. Your Green Beauty Smoothie will be ready for you to enjoy it.

2. Healthy Skin Berry Smoothie:

A cool looking smoothie that contains all the "winning ingredients"! The freshness of berries coupled with the taste of yoghurt and flaxseeds will surely have you captivated. And, there is no denying the fact that berries are like "ninjas" against oxidants and other unpleasant substances that are harmful for your skin.

Add these ingredients into your blender. Blend for about 2 minutes and then enjoy the smooth creamy drink.

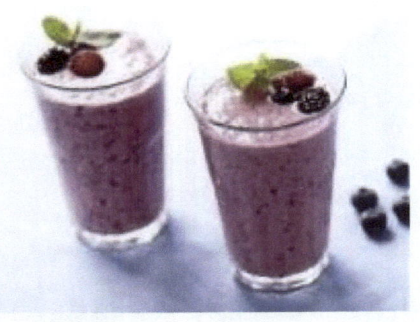

Ingredients

½ bowl of blueberries

¼ bowl of raspberries

¼ bowl of strawberries

¼ bowl of kale

1 fat free pack of yoghurt

1 TSP honey

2 TSP flax seeds

½ cup water

3. Coconut Water and Strawberry Smoothie:

Chilly coconut water, fresh strawberries and oranges… can't get better than that on a hot sunny day! The coconut water will keep your skin fresh by supporting the fatty acids beneath it and the strawberries will fulfill your vitamin C deficiency.

Add these things in your blender along with some ice to make a real smooth and chilly drink.

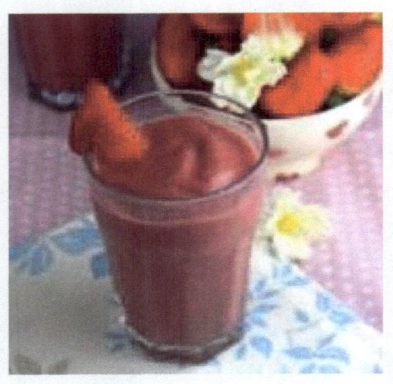

Ingredients

A cup of chilled coconut water

A small bowl of fresh strawberries

1 cup of organic carrots

A cup of fresh mango pieces

A peeled naval orange

4. Almond Banana Delight:

An unbelievably tasty and appetizing smoothie! It's a perfect combination of almonds and bananas that will prove to be a perfect start for a busy summer day.

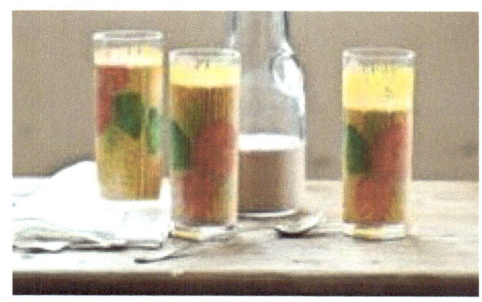

Blend all of these until you have yourself a smooth drink.

Ingredients

A frozen banana in small pieces'

1 TSP of peanut butter

2 TSP of flax seeds

½ cup of milk

A drizzle of maple syrup

A drop of almond or vanilla extract

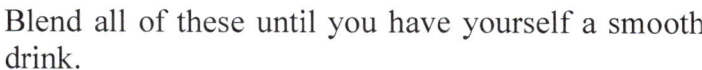

5. Berry Beauty Smoothie:

A beautiful and delectable combination of strawberries and blueberries that will have you hooked right away. These along with some other novel ingredients are the perfect skin cleansing tools.

Just blend until it gets smooth and enjoy it while relaxing, reading a novel or watching TV.

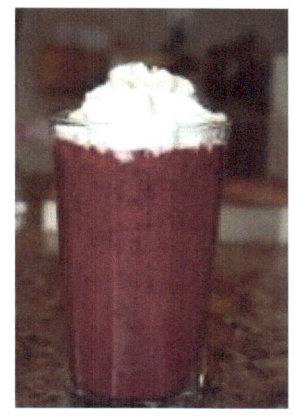

Ingredients

¼ cup of frozen strawberries and same quantity of blueberries

One peeled orange

A banana

½ cup of plain yoghurt

Silken tofu, ½ cup

2 TSP chia seeds and 1 TSP agave nectar

6. Superb Complexion Smoothie:

The usage of simple ingredients like kale and spinach gives this smoothie a great flavor and make it extremely healthy. Kale is a medically proven vegetable that helps in making your complexion fair. Besides kale, this smoothie is packed with loads of nutritious and scrumptious elements.

Put all the ingredients in your blender and blend at

slow speed for about 20 seconds. Then move to medium and high speed within the next 60 seconds. In less than 2 minutes, you'll have yourself a wonderful green smoothie.

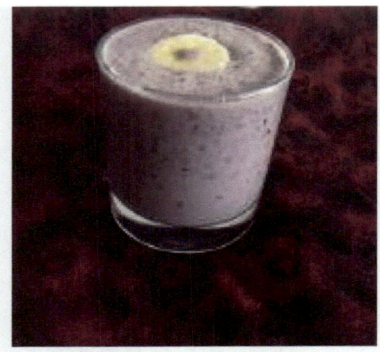

Ingredients

A cup of both spinach and kale leaves

A cup of green grapes

A pear with its seeds, core and stem removed

1 orange and 1 banana, both peeled

1 TSP chia seeds

½ cup of water

1 glass ice

7. Avocado Smoothie:

Composed of avocado and other fruits, this smoothie is loaded with vitamins E, C and K that are needed for maintaining healthy and fresh skin. And if you are suffering from skin inflammation, this smoothie is the right thing for you.

Puree all ingredients in your blender until smooth. Best to have it after a workout and replenish your lost minerals.

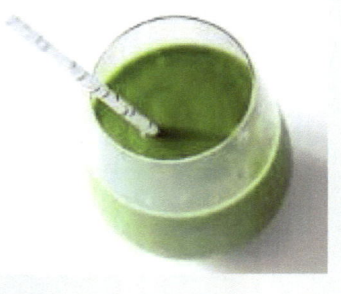

Ingredients

One ripe peach

Chopped Avocado, 2 tablespoon

4-5 frozen strawberries

About ½ cup of fat-free yoghurt

3 tsp pomegranate juice

Grape-seed oil and vanilla extract, 1 tsp each

C H A P T E R   8

Smoothie Recipes for Weight Loss

Achieving that perfect figure seems really hard…Think…think…what to do to reduce the undesired fat from your body? The answer is not that complicated. That's right! Don't worry about complex menus to reduce weight which don't really give the choice of good taste. Here is a variety of smoothies which are easy to make and are the best source to incorporate fresh fruits and vegetables. These smoothie recipes also provide you with the much needed monounsaturated fatty acids which aim to reduce belly fat. They are creamy, rich and perfect for breakfast, lunch or as a snack.

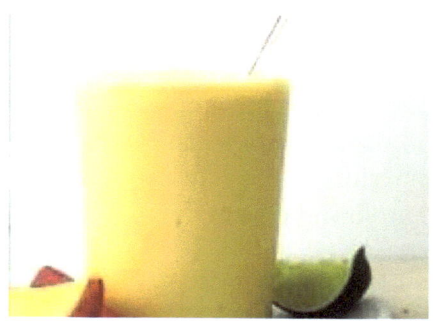

Ingredients

Mango cubes – 1/4 cup

Mango juice – 1/2 cup

Avocado – 1/4 cup

Fresh lime juice – 1 Tbsp

6 ice cubes

1. Mango Surprise

Who says that you need to completely cut out sweet flavors in order to reduce weight? This smoothie will satisfy your hunger for something sweet and at the same time reduce weight. Mangoes have high fiber and water content. That's why they not only help prevent constipation but fiber makes you feel full and satisfied for a long time. This is the key to reduce weight: take in a lot of fiber.

Process them in a blender and garnish with any fruit if you like.

2. Purple Smoothie

Blueberries are low on sugar content and rich in

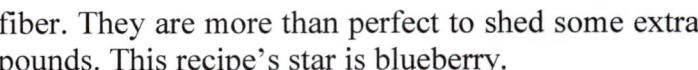

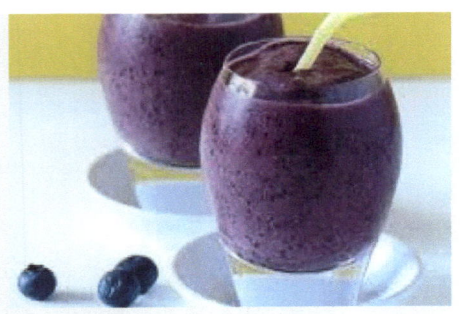

fiber. They are more than perfect to shed some extra pounds. This recipe's star is blueberry.

Blend blueberries and skim milk for 1 minute. Pour in the glass and mix the oil.

Ingredients

Unsweetened, frozen blueberries – 1 cup

Skim milk – 1 cup

Cold-pressed, organic flax seed oil – 1 Tbsp

3. Banana Boom

This amazing fruit is packed with all those superb nutrients to keep you smart and healthy. If combined with calcium rich foods like yoghurt and milk, you won't need anything else.

Combine all ingredients in a blender and process until it becomes a fine shake.

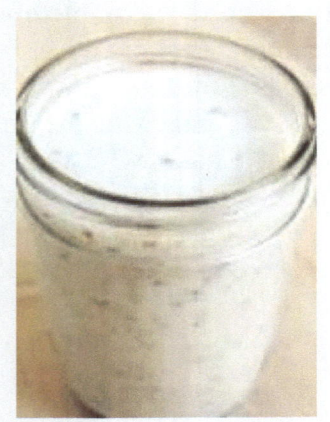

Ingredients

1 banana

Plain fat-free yoghurt – half cup

Fat-free milk – half cup

Unsalted peanut butter – 2 Tbsp

Honey- 1 Tbsp

4 ice cubes

4. Blueberry and Vanilla Yoghurt Smoothie

This smoothie is perfect for you to lose weight because it offers fiber, the richness of yoghurt and that amazing vanilla flavor. You won't miss your ice cream if you try this.

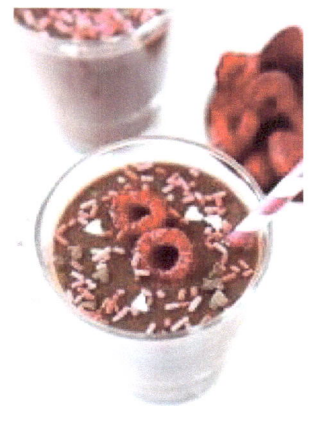

Ingredients

1 cup frozen blueberries

6 ounce vanilla yoghurt

1 cup skim milk

1 tablespoon flaxseed oil

Shake all the ingredients in a blender except flaxseed oil. When shaken properly, pour in a glass and mix the flaxseed oil.

5. Raspberry and Chocolate Smoothie

Huh! Chocolate! Well, don't be surprised. This isn't any sweet chocolate which will make you look like a bear. This smoothie recipe includes chocolate chips in a small quantity which will provide you with monounsaturated fatty acids i.e. the healthy fats. They will make your smoothie satisfying and help your body absorb vitamins.

Blend for 1 minute and relish this smoothie any time.

Ingredients

Fresh Raspberries – 1 cup

Chocolate chips – 1/4 cup

Skim milk – half cup

Vanilla yoghurt – 6 oz

Frozen raspberries – 1 cup

6. Peachy Shake

Refreshing and light, is what can be said about this smoothie. The main fruit in this recipe is perfect for achieving that ideal body weight and also give a fresh tone to your skin.

Always add flaxseed oil in the glass after shaking the ingredients. Such an easy way to become slim and smart!

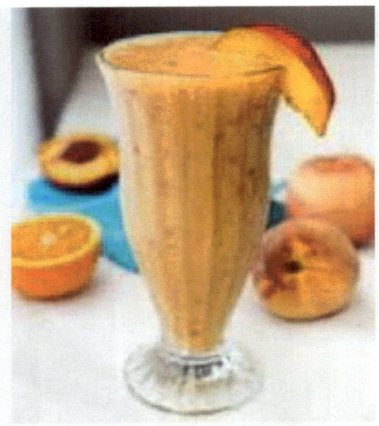

Ingredients

Frozen, unsweetened peaches – 1 cup

Skim milk – 1 cup

Cold-pressed organic flaxseed oil – 2 Tbsp

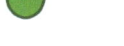

7. Citrus Smoothie

Citrus fruits such as orange and lemon are highly recommended when you are struggling to lose that stubborn body fat which makes you look older than your age.

Peel and section the orange and pop everything in the blender except the flaxseed oil. Add the oil after processing the ingredients. This smoothie will make you feel good.

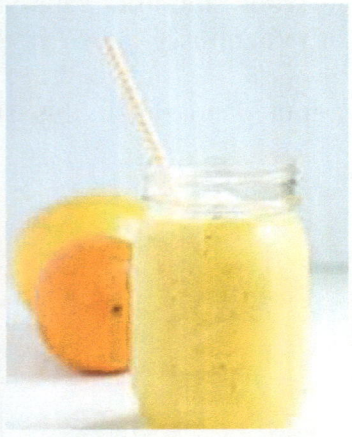

Ingredients

1 orange

Lemon Yoghurt – 6 oz

Skim milk – 1 cup

Flaxseed oil – 1 Tbsp

Some ice

C H A P T E R   9

Anti-Aging Smoothies

There are so many stories about the fountain of youth, how people tried to get there, and all that aura of romance surrounding these stories. While listening to and reading these stories some of you must have thought about that pure beauty and youth which catches the eye at once. Here is some news for you; you can make your own fountain of youth. That's right! There are some things which will slow down your aging process and make you look a lot younger. Anti-aging smoothies are that fountain of youth that you can make with some ingredients at the push of a button. Magic! Isn't it? These smoothies contain those ingredients which will improve your overall health and give your skin a nice glow. Here are some amazing recipes for you.

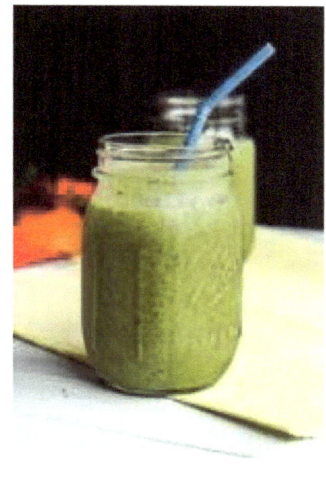

Ingredients

Blueberries – half cup

Strawberries – 1/4 cup

1 banana

1 orange

Tofu – half cup

Fat-free plain yoghurt – half cup

Agave nectar – 1 tsp

Chia seeds – 2 Tbsp

1. Healthy Beauty

This smoothie delivers a lot of vitamins, minerals and immune sytem boosting nutrients. Chia seeds, tofu and yoghurt provide you with calcium, proteins and iron to reduce inflammation and protect and maintain cell membranes. A+ Grade for the fruits because they help in building skin-firming collagen, rebuild skin cells and work against oxidative damage. Drink for health and beauty.

Prep all the fruits and whip all ingredients until smooth. Drink and think about regaining the splendor of youth.

2. Kale and Spinach Smoothie

The secret behind gorgeous skin – kale! It's full of carotenoids which gives your skin a healthy touch and makes it glow. Not only that, it also protects your skin from wrinkles. Drinking this smoothie is a perfect way to look attractive.

Chop kale, spinach and pear. Peel banana and orange and remove the seeds of orange. Place all the ingredients in Nutribullet and blend for 15 seconds. Then process until everything is nice and smooth.

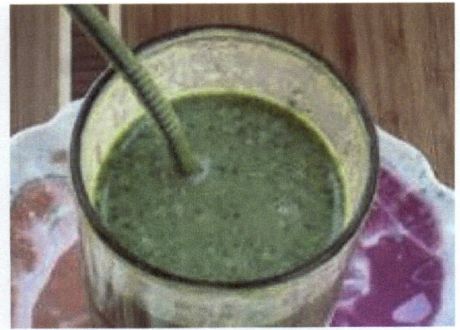

Ingredients

Kale – 1 cup

Spinach – 1cup

Green seedless grapes – 1cup

1 pear

1 banana

1 orange

Chia seeds – 1 tsp

Water – half cup

Ice – 2 cups

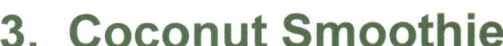

3. Coconut Smoothie

Beauty tips are not all about applying sun block, different cosmetics and even natural ingredients over your skin. There is no denying that these things help but you need something more. Something in the diet perhaps can help you gain awesome loveliness and heath at the same time. Including smoothies in your diet is the easiest way to look pretty. Coconut smoothie is one of the crucial drinks because coconut contains healthy fats. The presence of lauric acid in coconut oil gives it antimicrobial properties. Vitamin E in coconut is good for skin repair and growth. Last but not least, the saturated fat in coconut oil even protects the skin from UV damage. Include this amazing fruit in your smoothies and gain youth like beauty.

Blend all ingredients and enjoy the taste of youth.

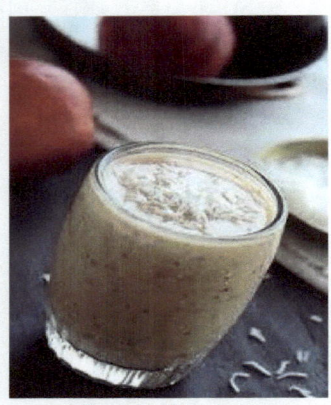

Ingredients

1 Sustain packet

Shredded unsweetened coconut – 1 Tbsp

Coconut oil – 1 Tbsp

Unsweetened almond milk – 4 oz

Water – 4 oz

Half banana

4 ice cubes

4. Avocado and Strawberry Smoothie

Here are the avocados! You must be thinking: "Yeah, what do they do?" and "What's the excitement for?" Let me tell you, they are loaded with vitamins C, E, and K which are very important for healthy skin. They also help in reducing dryness

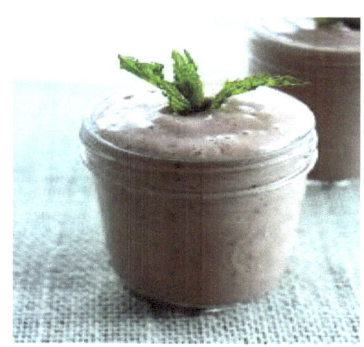

and irritation. Moreover, they contain glutathione which blocks intestinal absorption of certain fats that cause damage to the skin. Now what do you think?

Puree all ingredients well in a blender. It must be yummy.

Ingredients

Chopped Hass avocado – 2 Tbsp

1 peach

Unsweetened frozen strawberries – 1/3 cup

Pure pomegranate juice – 3 Tbsp

Fat-free plain yoghurt – 3/4 cup

Vanilla extract – 1 tsp

Grapeseed oil – 1 tsp

5. Berry Blast

It you want to make your skin perfect from the inside out, try some berries. Berries are packed with anti-oxidants which neutralize the free radicals that damage our skin cells. Hydrating water and vitamin C in the berries are essential for a healthy complexion. Do you want to know more? They also help the body manufacture collagen which gives your skin a flawless beauty.

Just crush these ingredients in your blender and get numerous benefits.

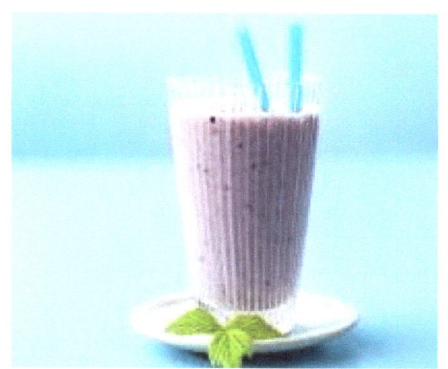

Ingredients

Raspberries – 1/4 cup

Blueberries – 1/4 cup

Strawberries – 1/4 cup

Kale – 1/4 cup

Water – 1 cup

6. Tropical Vacation

Composed of a lot of wonderful fruits, this smoothie will make you feel that you are on vacation in the Caribbean. Mango and pineapple in this smoothie will slow down the aging process because of vitamin C, beta carotene and omega 3.

Whirl them in your blender, take a sip and imagine the view of the beach…

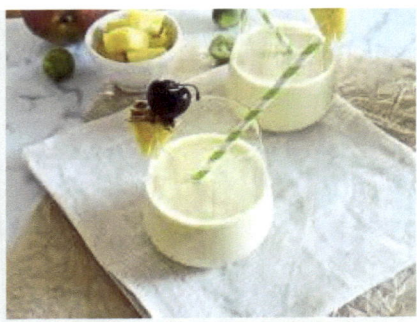

Ingredients

2 mangoes

Half pineapple

2 kiwis

Orange juice – 1 cup

3 ice cubes

7. Keep Me Active Smoothie

This smoothie will remove dark circles, keep you active and energetic. Must try!.

Hopefully, you'll appreciate the energetic punch of this smoothie.

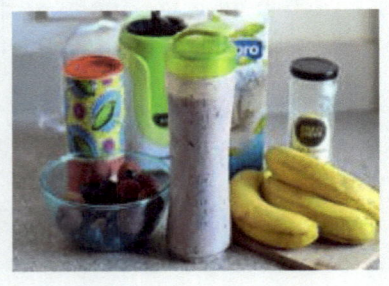

Ingredients

Blueberries – 1 cup

Raspberries – 2 cups

Flaxseed powder – 2 Tbsp

Goji berry powder – 1 Tbsp

Kefir – 1 cup

8. Fountain of Youth

This anti-aging smoothie will make you smart and healthy. Bananas in this smoothie will aid with digestion and green tea powder will keep you active, combat inflammation and reduce the risk of diseases because it contains polyphenols and caffeine. The coconut water and strawberries will illuminate your skin. How cool!

Combine all these beneficial ingredients and process in your blender. Your smoothie is ready.

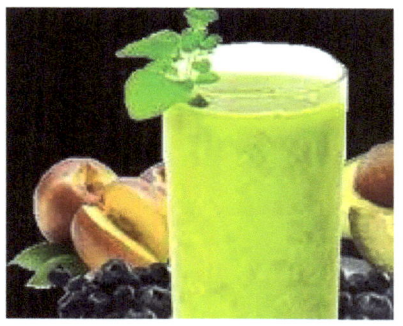

Ingredients

Strawberries – 3 cups

Green tea powder – 1 Tbsp

1 banana

Chia seed powder – 2 Tbsp

Coconut powder – 1 cup

C H A P T E R   1 0
Superfood Smoothies

We hear the term "superfoods" a lot these days but we don't really know what these are? Let me tell you that these foods are rich in nutrients that our bodies need but don't receive. The most common superfoods are chia seeds, flax seeds, coconut oil, spirulina, cacao nibs, avocado, hemp protein, camu powder and acai. A lot of us usually use these foods in meals and snacks but they can be used in smoothies as well. In fact, a smoothie composed of superfoods will boost up your stamina and make you really energetic.

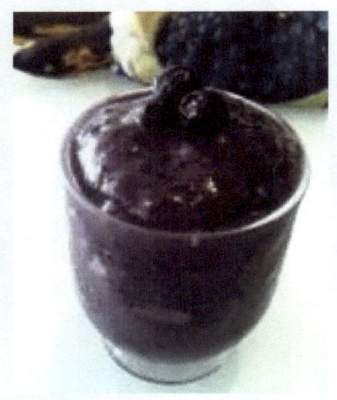

Ingredients

A cup of almond milk

Frozen blueberries, raspberries and soaked almonds, ¼ cup each

1 tablespoon butter

1 TSP cacao powder

Cinnamon and vanilla extract, ¼ tablespoon

1 TSP honey

1. Choco-Berry Almond Smoothie

It has chocolate, almond milk, blueberries and a bunch of other exciting ingredients which make it a worthy meal replacement.

Put these ingredients in your blender and blend for about 45 seconds. Add a few chunks of fresh strawberries along with some cacao nibs. Enjoy!!

2. The Dream Smoothie

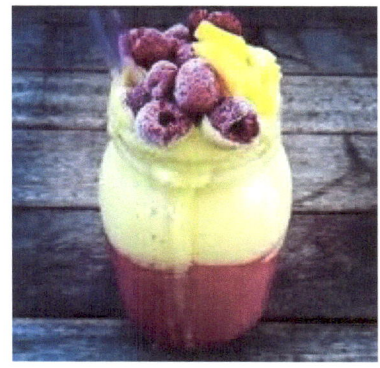

This recipe has all the dreamy ingredients. Avocado, blueberries, almonds, you name it! Whether you are exhausted after a harsh workout or drained after a long day at work, this smoothie will rock you up.

Blend all ingredients in your Nutribullet until smooth.

Ingredients

A cup of almond milk
½ cup fat-free yoghurt
½ piece of avocado
½ cup of blueberries, frozen preferably
2-3 Brazil nuts
1 TSP cacao powder
1 TSP cacao nibs
1 TSP maca
1 TSP lucuma
1/4 TSP cinnamon
2-3 drops of vanilla extract
A serving of protein powder of your choice

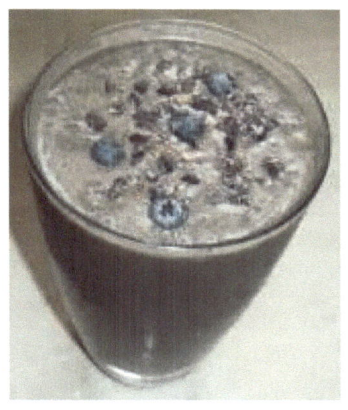

3. Spirulina with Chocolate and Blueberry Smoothie:

A real hardcore smoothie with a perfect combination of blueberries and spirulina! Now you can have your vitamins and minerals all in one glass of this smoothie.

Just blend all the ingredients until smooth and knock yourself out!

Ingredients

A cup of milk
One-third of an avocado
Half a cup of frozen blueberries
1 TSP of both tahini and cacao powder
½ TSP cacao nibs
½ TSP spirulina
½ TSP vanilla extract
½ TSP honey

4. Cacao Acai Smoothie

If you want to save yourself from cancer, premature aging and other kinds of nasty diseases, then grab your blender and follow this recipe right away. The acai and cacao nibs in this smoothie recipe are full of antioxidants that kill free radicals and other bad boys that may cause harm to your body.

Blend till smooth.

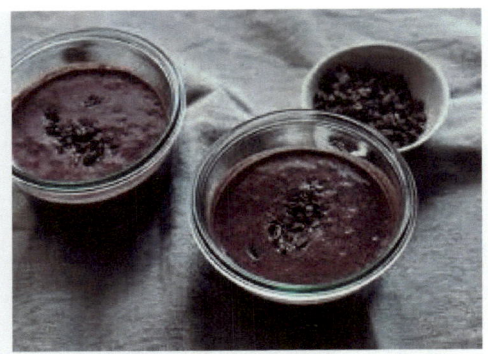

Ingredients

Coconut water, 1 cup

1/3 avocado

1/2 cup of yoghurt

1/2 cup of strawberries

1 TSP butter,

1 TSP cacao powder

1 TSP blended goji berries

Chia seeds, bee pollen and acai powder, 1 teaspoon each

1/4 teaspoon of cinnamon

A pinch of sea salt

1/2 tablespoon honey

5. Aloe Vera Citrus Smoothie

Aloe Vera is the champion of herbs because of its amazing medicinal characteristics. It helps in detoxification, improving immunity, digestion, countering inflammations and carcinogenic substances, skin freshness and above all it's a heart friendly herb. With so much to offer, it would be unwise not to use this splendid herb in a smoothie.

Add all the ingredients in your Nutribullet and blend for about 45 seconds. Pour it in a glass and garnish it with a peeled kiwi and half tablespoon of flax seeds.

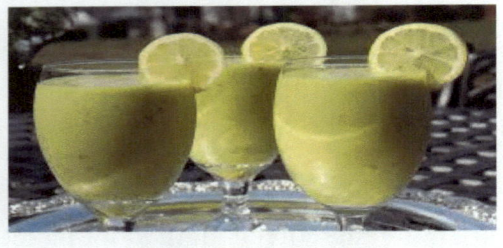

Ingredients

1 cup water

1/3 avocado

A medium sized aloe vera leaf

A small sized lemon, peeled

1 TSP coconut oil

A dash of salt

One tablespoon honey

4-5 ice cubes

6. Banana Delight Smoothie

Who doesn't like a creamy, scrummy banana smoothie on a hot summer eve? I wouldn't have second thoughts about not having it, would you? The chilly banana, fresh strawberries and mango chunks will make it difficult for you to stop.

Blend until smooth and let it cool you off!

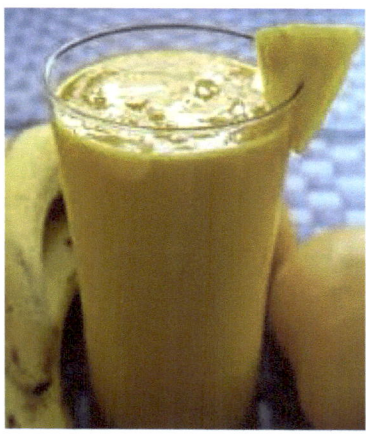

Ingredients

About 200g of almond milk

1 frozen banana

A cup of spinach

Frozen mango chunks and strawberries, 1/2 cup each

2 TSP Greek yoghurt

1 TSP coconut oil

1 TSP chia gel

1 TSP bee pollen

Conclusion

I hope this book was able to help you to make full use of your Nutribullet and prepare healthy and delicious smoothies and other meals.

The next step is to create a meal plan that will keep you motivated and dedicated to your fitness program.

The best thing about these recipes is that they only require some 'magical mixing' of ingredients and a little blending in your nutribullet and voila! Whether you need a smoothie to lose some extra pounds or you are looking for something to detoxify your body, the solution lies right here. The recipes include a whole bunch of healthy things like cinnamon, apples, oranges, broccoli, lime, blueberries, spinach etc. Everything has its unique advantage; some are known to burn down the 'troubling' layers of fats while others cleanse your body from all kinds of toxic stuff. There is good news for age conscious people as well. Now, you don't have to try any weird methods to slow down the process of aging

Did You Like Nutribullet Recipes?

Before you go, we'd like to say "thank you" for purchasing our book. So a big thanks for downloading this book and reading all the way to the end. Now we'd like ask for a *small* favor. Could you please take a minute or two and leave a review for this book on Amazon

This feedback will help us continue to write the kind of Kindle books that help you get results. And if you loved it, then please let me know

Leave a review for this book on Amazon by searching for the title **Nutribullet Recipes Lose Weight, Fight Aging, Gain Energy, and Improve Overall Health with the Superfood Detox Cleanse Smoothies**

Check Out My Other Books

Below you'll find some of my other popular books that are popular on Amazon and Kindle as well. Simply click on the links below to check them out. Alternatively, you can visit my author page on Amazon to see other work done by me.

amazon.com/author/jjlewis

101 Pork Chop Recipes: Extraordinary and Delicious Pork Chop Recipes for Everyday Meals

101 Chicken Recipes: A Mouth-Watering Healthy and Delicious Chicken Recipes that will fill your Stomach

101 Vegetarian Recipes: Top Vegan Diet Recipes to Live a Healthy Lifestyle

The Juice Cleanse: 101 Healthy Juicing Recipes for Weight Loss

Diabetes Diet: 101 Healthy Diabetes Recipes to Reverse Diabetes Forever and Enjoy Healthy Living for Life

Low Fat Recipes: 101 Incredible Quick & Easy Recipes for a Low Fat Diet

Gluten Free Diet: 101 Delectable and Healthy Gluten-Free Recipes for better lifestyle

Paleo Diet for Kids: A Fun Pack of 101 Flavorful and Energy-Boosting Paleo Recipes Best In Shaping Healthier, Stronger and Happier Paleo-Nourished Kids

Mediterranean Slow Cooker: 101 Best of Easy and Delicious Mediterranean Slow Cooker Recipes to a Healthy Life

Slow Cooker Recipes: The Best of 101 Nutritious and Delicious Healthy Slow-Cooking Recipes for your Crock Pot

Pressure Cooker Recipes: 101 Mouthwatering, Delicious, Easy and Healthy Pressure Cooker Recipes for Breakfast, Lunch, Dinner in 30 Minutes or Less!

Wheat Belly Diet: 101 Days of Grain Free Recipes for an Optimum Belly Diet and Weight Loss

Fast Metabolism Diet Recipes: 101 Best of Metabolism Boosting Recipes to Lose Weight Fast

You can simply search for these titles on the Amazon website to find them.

Want more Bestseller Cook Books for FREE?

Join my **V.I.P** Reading List where I give away **Healthy** and Delicious Recipes FOR **FREE!**

Yes, you heard me right! COMPLETELY FREE to everyone just for being a loyal reader of mine!

http://www.mritchi.com/freecookbook

www.ingramcontent.com/pod-product-compliance
Lightning Source LLC
Chambersburg PA
CBHW041518280526

45792CB00004B/1295